PROFESSIONAL MAKEUP FOR WOMEN

Pseudonym
Christopher Baldwin Heritage Blend

Sr. Gonzalo I Linares Amezcua

IA GENERATIVE OPENAI

ISBN: 9798326233042

Sello: Independently published

Contouring and Highlighting: Defining and enhancing facial features

Facial Corrections: Camouflaging dark circles, blemishes, imperfections, and asymmetries

Makeup Setting: Techniques to keep your look impeccable all day long

Part 3: Makeup for Special Occasions

Daytime Makeup: Natural and sophisticated looks for daytime events

Evening Makeup: Glamorous and elegant styles for special occasions

Smoky Eye Makeup: Techniques to create an intense and mysterious look

Dramatic Eye Makeup: Application of false eyelashes, graphic liners, and vibrant colors

Statement Lip Makeup: Red lips, ombre, and special effects

Makeup for Social Events: Weddings, graduations, parties, and celebrations

Themed Makeup: Carnival, Halloween, costume parties

Part 4: Advanced Makeup and Special Effects

High-Definition Makeup: Professional techniques for a flawless finish on camera and events

Advanced Contouring: Extreme facial definition, sculpted cheekbones, and profiled noses

Strobing: Strategic highlighting for a radiant and vibrant look

3D Makeup: Creating volume and dimension on the face using advanced techniques

Artistic Makeup: Character design, special effects, and creative transformations

Makeup for Mature Skin: Tips and techniques to enhance beauty at all ages

Makeup for Different Ethnicities: Considerations and tips for adapting makeup to every skin tone

Part 5: Professional Makeup Aspects

Hygiene and Sanitization: Essential practices for a professional and safe work environment

Ethics and Professionalism: Values and fundamental principles in the makeup industry

Marketing and Personal Promotion: Creating a personal brand and strategies to attract clients

Business Management: Organization, administration, and customer service in a makeup studio

Makeup Trends: Analysis of the latest trends and their professional application

Runway and Editorial Makeup: Techniques and styles for the fashion world

Film and Television Makeup: Characterization and demands of the audiovisual medium

Special Effects Makeup: Creating prosthetics, wounds, and realistic transformations

Part 6: Resources and Supplements

Glossary of Terms: Definitions of key words and relevant concepts in the world of makeup

Recommended Products and Brands: Guide to selecting high-quality makeup products

Inspiration and References: Artists, trends, and styles to broaden your creativity

Online Resources: Tutorials, blogs, and learning platforms to keep improving

Practice and Experimentation: The key to mastering techniques and developing your own style

Passion and Dedication: The essential ingredient for success in a professional makeup career

Professional Makeup Book for Women: A Comprehensive Guide to Mastering the Art of Makeup

Anatomy of the Face and Color Theory Understanding the anatomy of the face is crucial for mastering the art of makeup. By knowing the structure of the face, you can enhance its natural beauty and create a flawless look. In this chapter, we will explore the different features of the face and how to highlight them through makeup techniques. We will also delve into color theory and how it applies to makeup. By understanding the color wheel and how different shades complement each other, you can create harmonious and balanced looks. Whether you have warm or cool undertones, knowing how to choose the right tones for your skin will make a world of difference in your makeup application. Throughout this chapter, you will learn the fundamentals of skincare and how to prepare your canvas for makeup application. From cleansing and moisturizing to priming and setting, taking care of your skin is essential for achieving a flawless makeup look. By the end of this chapter, you will have a solid foundation in the anatomy of the face and color theory, setting the stage for the rest of the book as we dive into more advanced makeup techniques. Get ready to unleash your creativity and master the art of makeup like a true professional.

Part 1: Makeup Fundamentals

Makeup Fundamentals Welcome to the exciting world of makeup artistry! In this chapter, we will cover the essential fundamentals that every makeup artist should know in order to create beautiful and flawless looks. From understanding the anatomy of the face to mastering color theory, these basics will serve as the building blocks for your career in makeup. Anatomy of the Face: Before diving into the world of makeup, it is crucial to have a good understanding of the anatomy of the face. Knowing the different features of the face, such as the eyes, nose, lips, and cheekbones, will help you determine the best techniques to enhance and accentuate each area. By familiarizing yourself with the structure of the face, you will be able to create balanced and harmonious looks that highlight your client's natural beauty. Colorimetry: Color theory plays a significant role in makeup artistry, as it helps you choose the right tones and shades to complement your client's skin tone. Understanding the color wheel and how different colors interact with each other will enable you to create harmonious and flattering makeup looks. Whether you are selecting foundation shades, eyeshadows, or lip colors, having a solid grasp of color theory will elevate your makeup artistry skills to the next level. Basic and Advanced Makeup Techniques: In this chapter, we will cover a range of basic and advanced makeup techniques for the eyes, lips, and face. From creating a flawless base with foundation and concealer to mastering the art of eyeshadow blending and lipstick application, these techniques will help you achieve professional-looking results. Whether you are a beginner or an experienced makeup artist, mastering these fundamental techniques is essential for creating stunning makeup looks. Tricks and Tips for Different Occasions: As a makeup artist, you will encounter a variety of clients with different preferences and needs. In this chapter, we will share tricks and tips for creating natural looks, daytime makeup, evening makeup, special occasion looks, and themed event makeup. Whether you are attending a wedding, a red carpet event, or a costume party, having the knowledge and skills to adapt your makeup techniques to suit the occasion is crucial for success in the industry. Professional Makeup Techniques: To take your makeup artistry skills to the next level, we will delve into professional techniques such as high definition makeup, contouring, strobing, and 3D makeup. These advanced techniques are used in the world of film, television, and fashion to create stunning and impactful makeup looks. By mastering these techniques, you will be able to offer your clients a wide range of services and stand out as a professional makeup artist in the industry. Ethical, Business, and Marketing Aspects: In addition to mastering the art of makeup, it is essential to understand the ethical, business, and marketing aspects of being a professional makeup artist. In this chapter, we will cover topics such as client confidentiality, hygiene practices, pricing your services, building a portfolio, and marketing yourself as a makeup artist. By understanding these crucial aspects of the industry, you will be able to build a successful and sustainable career as a makeup artist. Resources and Complements: To continue expanding your knowledge and skills as a makeup artist, it is important to have access to a range of resources and complements. In this chapter, we will provide recommendations for books, online courses, workshops, and networking opportunities that will help you stay up-to-date with the latest trends and techniques in the world of makeup artistry. By investing in your education and continuously learning and growing as a makeup artist, you will be able to reach new heights of success in your career. In conclusion, mastering the fundamentals of makeup artistry is essential for becoming a successful and professional makeup artist. By understanding the anatomy of the face, color theory, basic and advanced makeup techniques, tricks and tips for different occasions, professional makeup techniques, ethical, business, and marketing aspects, and resources and complements, you will be well-equipped to excel in this exciting and dynamic industry. Stay tuned for the next chapter, where we will dive deeper into the world of makeup artistry and explore advanced techniques and trends in the field.

Facial Anatomy: Zones, proportions, and key features

Facial Anatomy: Zones, Proportions, and Key Features
Understanding facial anatomy is essential for any

professional makeup artist. By knowing the different zones of the face, their proportions, and key features, you will be able to enhance your client's natural beauty and create flawless makeup looks. Zones of the Face: The face can be divided into several zones, each with its own characteristics and features. These zones include the forehead, eyebrows, eyes, nose, cheeks, lips, chin, and jawline. By understanding the unique qualities of each zone, you can create balanced and harmonious makeup looks that accentuate your client's best features. Proportions: Proportions play a key role in makeup application, as they help create symmetry and balance on the face. The golden ratio, also known as the rule of thirds, can be used to determine the ideal proportions for the eyes, eyebrows, nose, and lips. By following these proportions, you can create a harmonious and visually pleasing makeup look that enhances your client's natural beauty. Key Features: Every face has its own unique features that should be accentuated through makeup application. Key features such as high cheekbones, full lips, and defined eyebrows can be enhanced using contouring, highlighting, and other advanced makeup techniques. By focusing on these key features, you can create a personalized makeup look that highlights your client's best assets. In this chapter, we will delve deeper into the anatomy of the face, exploring the different zones, proportions, and key features that makeup artists should be aware of. By mastering these fundamental concepts, you will be able to create stunning makeup looks that enhance your client's natural beauty and leave them feeling confident and beautiful.

Color Theory: Harmonies, contrasts, and applications in makeup

Color Theory: Harmonies, Contrasts, and Applications in Makeup Understanding color theory is essential for any professional makeup artist. By mastering the principles of harmonies and contrasts, you can create stunning looks that enhance your client's natural beauty. Harmonies: Harmonious color combinations are pleasing to the eye and create a sense of balance in makeup looks. The most common harmonies used in makeup include: - Monochromatic: using shades of the same color for a subtle and cohesive look. - Analogous: combining colors that are next to each other on the color wheel for a harmonious effect. - Complementary: pairing colors that are opposite each other on the color wheel for a bold and striking look. Contrasts: Contrasting colors can create drama and interest in makeup looks. Some popular contrasts to consider include: - Warm vs. Cool: mixing warm tones (reds, oranges, yellows) with cool tones (blues, greens, purples) for a dynamic look. - Light vs. Dark: using light shades to highlight and dark shades to contour and define features. - Matte vs. Shimmer: playing with different finishes to add dimension and depth to the makeup look. Applications: Once you understand color theory, you can apply these principles to create a wide variety of makeup looks. Some popular applications include: - Smokey Eye: using contrasting shades to create a sultry and smoldering eye look. - Bold Lip: pairing a bold lip color with neutral eye makeup for a statement look. - Color Blocking: using contrasting colors on different areas of the face for a modern and edgy look. Experimenting with different color combinations and techniques will help you develop your own unique style as a makeup artist. Remember to consider your client's skin tone, eye color, and personal preferences when choosing colors for their makeup look. By mastering color theory, you can elevate your makeup skills and create beautiful looks that will leave your clients feeling confident and glamorous. Keep practicing and experimenting with different colors to expand your knowledge and skills as a professional makeup artist.

Skin Care: Cleansing, moisturizing, sun protection, and makeup prep

Skin Care: Cleansing, moisturizing, sun protection, and makeup prep In order to achieve flawless makeup application, it is essential to start with a clean and well-prepped canvas. Skin care plays a crucial role in ensuring that your makeup looks smooth, radiant, and long-lasting. In this chapter, we will delve into the importance of cleansing, moisturizing, sun protection, and makeup prep in achieving the perfect makeup look. Cleansing: The first step in any skincare routine is cleansing. Cleansing helps to remove dirt, oil, and makeup residue from the skin, allowing for better absorption of skincare products and makeup. Choose a gentle cleanser that is suitable for your skin type, whether it be dry, oily, combination, or sensitive. Use lukewarm water to avoid stripping the skin of its natural oils, and pat dry with a clean towel. Moisturizing: Moisturizing is key to maintaining healthy and hydrated skin. Choose a moisturizer that suits your skin type and concerns, whether it be lightweight for oily skin, rich for dry skin, or containing SPF for added sun protection. Apply moisturizer in gentle upward strokes, focusing on areas that tend to be dry or prone to fine lines. Sun Protection: Sun protection is crucial in preventing premature aging and skin damage. Always apply a broad-spectrum sunscreen with at least SPF 30 before stepping out into the sun, even on cloudy days. Reapply every two hours, especially if you are sweating or swimming. Opt for a lightweight, non-comedogenic formula that won't clog pores or interfere with your makeup. Makeup Prep: Before applying makeup, it is important to prime the skin to create a smooth and even base. Use a makeup primer that addresses your specific concerns, whether it be minimizing pores, controlling oil, or adding radiance. Apply primer evenly all over the face, focusing on areas where makeup tends to crease or fade. By incorporating proper skin care practices into your makeup routine, you can ensure that your makeup looks flawless and lasts throughout the day. Remember, beautiful makeup starts with healthy skin. Stay tuned for the next chapter, where we will dive into the world of color theory and how to choose the perfect shades for your skin tone.

Tools and Brushes: Types, uses, and care of essential makeup instruments

Tools and Brushes: Types, uses, and care of essential makeup instruments In the world of makeup, having the right tools and brushes is essential for achieving flawless and professional results. In this chapter, we will explore the different types of tools and brushes available, their uses, and how to properly care for them to ensure longevity and effectiveness. Types of Tools and Brushes 1. Foundation Brushes: Used to apply liquid or cream foundation evenly onto the skin. There are different shapes and sizes available, such as flat, angled, and stippling brushes. 2. Concealer Brushes: Designed to target specific areas for concealing imperfections, such as blemishes or dark circles. These brushes are smaller and more precise than foundation brushes. 3. Powder Brushes: Used to apply loose or pressed powder to set makeup and mattify the skin. These brushes come in various shapes, such as round, flat, or angled. 4. Eyeshadow Brushes: Essential for applying and blending eyeshadow colors. There are different types of eyeshadow brushes, such as flat shader brushes, blending brushes, and crease brushes. 5. Blush Brushes: Used to apply blush to the apples of the cheeks for a natural flush of color. These brushes are typically round or angled for precise application. 6. Lip Brushes: Ideal for applying lipstick or lip gloss with precision and control. Lip brushes are typically small and flat for easy application. Care of Essential Makeup Instruments To ensure the longevity and effectiveness of your makeup tools and brushes, it is important to properly care for them. Here are some tips for maintaining your essential makeup instruments: 1. Clean your brushes regularly: Makeup brushes can harbor bacteria and product buildup, so it is important to clean them at least once a week. Use a gentle brush cleaner or baby shampoo to remove dirt and makeup residue. 2. Store your tools properly: Keep your brushes and tools in a clean and dry place to prevent contamination and damage. Consider investing in a brush holder or organizer to keep them organized and protected. 3. Replace old or damaged brushes: Over time, makeup brushes can wear out or become damaged, leading to less effective application. Replace any brushes that are shedding bristles or no longer perform well. By understanding the different types of tools and brushes available, their uses, and how to properly care for them, you will be equipped to achieve professional and flawless makeup looks. Mastering the art of makeup requires not only skill and technique but also the right tools to bring your vision to life.

Makeup Products: Classification, characteristics, and selection based on skin type and needs

Makeup Products: Classification, characteristics, and selection based on skin type and needs In this chapter, we will delve into the world of makeup products, exploring their different classifications, characteristics, and how to select the right products based on skin type and individual needs. Understanding the various types of makeup products available in the market is essential for achieving flawless and long-lasting makeup looks. Classification of Makeup Products: 1. Foundation: Foundation is the base of any makeup look, providing coverage and evening out the skin tone. There are different types of foundations available, including liquid, cream, powder, and stick foundations. It is important to choose a foundation that matches your skin tone and type for a seamless finish. 2. Concealer: Concealer is used to hide imperfections such as dark circles, blemishes, and redness. It comes in various forms, including liquid, cream, and stick concealers. Select a concealer that is one shade lighter than your foundation for a brightening effect. 3. Powder: Setting powder is used to set foundation and concealer, ensuring a matte finish and helping makeup last longer. Loose and pressed powders are popular choices, with translucent powders being ideal for all skin tones. 4. Blush: Blush adds a pop of color to the cheeks, enhancing the overall makeup look. There are different types of blushes, including powder, cream, and liquid formulas. Choose a blush shade that complements your skin tone for a natural flush. 5. Eyeshadow: Eyeshadow comes in a variety of finishes, including matte, shimmer, and metallic. It is essential to select eyeshadow shades that complement your eye color and skin tone for a cohesive look. Primer can be used to enhance the vibrancy and longevity of eyeshadow. 6. Mascara: Mascara is used to lengthen, volumize, and define the lashes. Choose a mascara formula that suits your desired lash look, whether it be lengthening, volumizing, or curling. 7. Lipstick: Lipstick adds color and definition to the lips, completing the makeup look. There are various lipstick finishes, including matte, satin, and gloss. Select a lipstick shade that complements your skin tone and outfit. Selection Based on Skin Type and Needs: When selecting makeup products, it is important to consider your skin type and individual needs. For oily skin, opt for oil-free and matte products to control shine. Dry skin benefits from hydrating and creamy formulas to prevent flakiness. Combination skin requires products that balance oil and hydration. Additionally, consider any skin concerns you may have, such as acne, sensitivity, or aging. Look for products that are non-comedogenic, fragrance-free, and anti-aging to address these concerns effectively. Experiment with different products and techniques to find what works best for your skin type and needs. Remember to always remove makeup thoroughly at the end of the day to maintain healthy skin. By understanding the classification, characteristics, and selection of makeup products based on skin type and needs, you can achieve flawless and personalized makeup looks. Experiment with different products and techniques to enhance your natural beauty and express your unique style.

Lighting and Colorimetry: Techniques for proper lighting and makeup shade selection

Lighting and Colorimetry: Techniques for proper lighting and makeup shade selection In the world of professional makeup, lighting plays a crucial role in achieving flawless results. Understanding how different types of lighting affect the way makeup looks on the skin is essential for any makeup artist. In this chapter, we will delve into the importance of proper lighting and colorimetry in makeup application. Colorimetry is the science of color and how it is perceived by the human eye. When it comes to makeup, choosing the right shades for your skin tone is key to creating a harmonious and natural look. Understanding the color wheel and how different colors interact with each other will help you select the perfect shades for your clients. Proper lighting is essential for achieving the best results in makeup application. Natural light is the most flattering for makeup as it mimics the conditions in which makeup is usually worn. When applying makeup, it is important to have a well-lit area with natural light to ensure that you are able to see the true colors of the products you are using. When working in artificial lighting, it is important to be aware of the different types of lighting and how they can affect the way makeup looks on the skin. Fluorescent lighting can make makeup appear more yellow or green, while incandescent lighting can make makeup appear more pink or red. It is important to adjust your makeup application accordingly to ensure that your client looks their best in any lighting situation. When selecting makeup shades, it is important to consider the undertones of your client's skin. Warm undertones look best in golden or peachy tones, while cool undertones look best in pink or blue-based shades. Understanding how undertones work will help you choose the right shades for your clients and create a seamless and natural look. In this chapter, we will also discuss techniques for proper makeup shade selection and how to adjust your makeup application based on the lighting conditions. By mastering the art of lighting and colorimetry, you will be able to create stunning makeup looks that enhance your client's natural beauty and leave them feeling confident and beautiful.

Part 2: Basic Makeup Techniques

Part 2: Basic Makeup Techniques In this section of the Professional Makeup for Women manual, we will delve into the essential techniques every makeup artist should master. Whether you are a beginner looking to enhance your skills or a seasoned professional wanting to refine your craft, this chapter will provide you with the foundational knowledge needed to create stunning makeup looks. Anatomy of the Face and Colorimetry Understanding the anatomy of the face is crucial for creating a harmonious and balanced makeup look. By knowing the different facial features and their proportions, you can enhance your client's natural beauty and correct any imperfections. Additionally, colorimetry plays a key role in choosing the right tones for your client's skin. Learning how to identify undertones and select the appropriate foundation, concealer, and color products will ensure a flawless and cohesive makeup application. Application of Basic and Advanced Makeup Techniques From enhancing the eyes to defining the lips and sculpting the face, mastering basic makeup techniques is essential for creating a polished and professional look. In this section, we will cover everything from applying foundation and concealer to blending eyeshadow and creating a perfect winged eyeliner. Additionally, we will explore advanced techniques such as contouring, strobing, and 3D makeup, which can elevate your makeup game to the next level. Tricks and Tips for Different Occasions Whether you are creating a natural daytime look, a glamorous evening look, or a bold makeup look for a themed event, knowing the right tricks and tips can make all the difference. In this chapter, we will share insider secrets on how to achieve flawless makeup looks for any occasion. From choosing the right colors to creating long-lasting and smudge-proof makeup, you will learn how to cater to your client's preferences and enhance their natural beauty. Professional Makeup Techniques As a professional makeup artist, it is important to stay up-to-date with the latest trends and techniques in the industry. In this section, we will explore high-definition makeup, contouring, strobing, and 3D makeup, which are essential skills for creating camera-ready looks. By mastering these advanced techniques, you can offer your clients a flawless and sculpted appearance that will make them stand out from the crowd. Ethical, Business, and Marketing Aspects Becoming a successful professional makeup artist goes beyond mastering makeup techniques. In this chapter, we will discuss the ethical considerations, business strategies, and marketing tactics that are essential for building a thriving makeup artistry career. From maintaining client confidentiality to pricing your services competitively and promoting your brand effectively, you will learn how to navigate the business side of the industry with confidence. Resources and Complements To excel in the world of makeup artistry, it is important to continuously expand your knowledge and skills. In this final section, we will provide you with valuable resources, such as books, courses, and online platforms, where you can further your education and stay inspired. Additionally, we will recommend complementary services, such as skincare treatments and beauty consultations, that can enhance your makeup services and provide a holistic approach to beauty. By mastering the basic makeup techniques outlined in this chapter and incorporating advanced techniques into your repertoire, you will be well on your way to becoming a professional makeup artist. With dedication, practice, and a passion for beauty, you can create stunning makeup looks that enhance your client's natural features and boost their confidence. Stay inspired, stay creative, and never stop learning in this fascinating world of makeup artistry.

Natural Makeup: A fresh and radiant look for everyday wear

Natural Makeup: A fresh and radiant look for everyday wear In this chapter, we will delve into the world of natural makeup, a versatile and timeless look that enhances your features while still looking effortlessly beautiful. Whether you're heading to work, running errands, or meeting friends for lunch, natural makeup is the perfect choice for any occasion. Anatomy of the face and colorimetry play a crucial role in achieving a natural makeup look. Understanding the shape of your face and the undertones of your skin will help you choose the correct tones and products to enhance your natural beauty. Remember, the key to natural makeup is to enhance, not overpower. When it comes to applying natural makeup, less is more. Start by prepping your skin with a moisturizer and primer to create a smooth canvas. Use a light coverage foundation or BB cream to even out your skin tone, followed by a concealer to cover any imperfections. Opt for neutral eyeshadows, a hint of blush, and a natural lip color to complete your look. Tricks and tips are essential when it comes to creating a natural makeup look. For a fresh and radiant complexion, try using a cream blush for a natural flush of color. Curl your lashes and apply a coat of mascara to open up your eyes. To add a touch of glow, use a highlighter on the high points of your face, such as your cheekbones and brow bones. Natural makeup is all about enhancing your features and embracing your natural beauty. By mastering the art of natural makeup, you can achieve a fresh and radiant look for everyday wear that will leave you feeling confident and beautiful. Stay tuned for the next chapter where we will explore professional makeup techniques for high definition, contouring, strobing, and 3D makeup to take your skills to the next level.

Eye Makeup: Applying eyeshadows, eyeliners, mascara, and eyebrow shaping

Eye Makeup: Applying eyeshadows, eyeliners, mascara, and eyebrow shaping In this chapter, we will delve into the world of eye makeup, exploring the different techniques and products that can enhance the natural beauty of your eyes. From choosing the right eyeshadows to mastering the art of applying eyeliner and mascara, you will learn how to create stunning eye looks for any occasion. Eyeshadows are a versatile tool that can be used to add depth and dimension to your eyes. When applying eyeshadow, it's important to consider your eye shape and color to choose the most flattering shades. Start by applying a neutral base color all over the lid, then use a darker shade in the crease to add definition. Finish off with a light shimmer shade on the brow bone to highlight the eyes. Eyeliners come in a variety of forms, including pencil, gel, and liquid. Each type has its own unique application technique, so experiment with different formulas to find the one that works best for you. To apply eyeliner, start by drawing a thin line along the upper lash line, then extend it slightly beyond the outer corner for a winged effect. For a more dramatic look, you can also line the lower lash line. Mascara is a must-have product for adding volume and length to your lashes. When applying mascara, start at the base of the lashes and wiggle the wand back and forth to coat each lash evenly. For extra volume, apply multiple coats, focusing on the outer lashes for a flirty, winged effect. Eyebrows play a crucial role in framing the eyes and defining your facial features. To shape your eyebrows, start by brushing them upwards to reveal their natural shape. Use a brow pencil or powder to fill in any sparse areas, then use a spoolie brush to blend the color for a natural finish. Finish off with a clear brow gel to set the hairs in place. By mastering the art of eye makeup, you can enhance your natural beauty and create stunning looks for any occasion. Experiment with different techniques and products to find what works best for you, and don't be afraid to try new trends and styles. With practice and patience, you can become a pro at eye makeup and wow everyone with your stunning eye looks.

Lip Makeup: Outlining, filling, and techniques for different styles

Lip Makeup: Outlining, filling, and techniques for different styles Lips are an essential part of any makeup look, as they can instantly enhance and define the face. In this chapter, we will delve into the art of lip makeup, covering everything from outlining and filling to techniques for different styles. 1. Lip Outlining: Before applying any lip color, it is crucial to outline the lips to create a defined shape. Use a lip liner that matches the natural color of your lips or the lipstick you will be using. Start by outlining the cupid's bow and then move on to the corners of the mouth. For a fuller look, slightly overline the lips, staying close to the natural lip line to avoid a harsh appearance. 2. Lip Filling: Once you have outlined the lips, it's time to fill them in with your chosen lip color. Whether you prefer a matte, satin, or glossy finish, make sure to apply the lipstick evenly across the lips. You can use a lip brush for precision or apply directly from the bullet for a quicker application. Blot the lips with a tissue to remove any excess product and ensure long-lasting wear. 3. Techniques for Different Styles: There are endless possibilities when it comes to lip makeup styles. From classic red lips to trendy ombré effects, here are some techniques to experiment with: - Ombré Lips: Start by applying a darker shade on the outer corners of the lips and a lighter shade in the center. Blend the two colors together for a seamless gradient effect. - Glossy Lips: For a shiny finish, apply a clear lip gloss over your favorite lipstick. This will add dimension and make the lips appear plumper. - Bold Lips: Don't be afraid to rock a bold lip color, such as vibrant pink or deep plum. Pair it with minimal eye makeup for a statement look. - Nude Lips: Nude lip colors are perfect for a natural makeup look. Choose a shade that complements your skin tone and enhances your features. Experiment with different techniques and styles to find what works best for you. Remember to practice and have fun with lip makeup, as it can truly transform your overall look. In this chapter, we have covered the basics of lip makeup, including outlining, filling, and techniques for different styles. By mastering these techniques, you will be able to create a variety of lip looks to suit any occasion. Stay tuned for more advanced lip makeup tips and tricks in the following chapters.

Contouring and Highlighting: Defining and enhancing facial features

Contouring and Highlighting: Defining and Enhancing Facial Features Contouring and highlighting are essential techniques in the world of professional makeup. These techniques help define and enhance the natural features of the face, creating a more sculpted and radiant look. In this chapter, we will explore the art of contouring and highlighting, and how to master these techniques to elevate your makeup skills to the next level. Anatomy of the Face and Colorimetry Before delving into contouring and highlighting, it is important to understand the anatomy of the face and colorimetry. Understanding the structure of the face will help you identify the areas that can benefit from contouring and highlighting, while colorimetry will help you choose the correct tones for your skin. Application of Basic and Advanced Makeup Techniques Contouring and highlighting are advanced makeup techniques that require precision and skill. In this chapter, we will guide you through the step-by-step process of contouring and highlighting different facial features, such as the cheekbones, nose, and jawline. We will also explore how to blend these techniques seamlessly for a natural and flawless finish. Tricks and Tips for Different Looks Whether you are creating a natural everyday look or a glamorous evening look, contouring and highlighting can be tailored to suit any occasion. In this chapter, we will share tricks and tips for creating different makeup looks, including day, night, special occasions, and themed events. You will learn how to enhance your features to create a look that is uniquely yours. Professional Makeup Techniques Contouring and highlighting are not just limited to traditional makeup. In this chapter, we will explore professional techniques such as high definition makeup, strobing, and 3D makeup.

These techniques are used in photography, film, and television to create a flawless and dimensional look. By mastering these techniques, you will be able to create stunning makeup looks that stand out on camera. Ethical, Business, and Marketing Aspects Becoming a successful professional makeup artist requires more than just skill and talent. In this chapter, we will discuss the ethical, business, and marketing aspects of the industry. From building a portfolio to networking with clients, we will guide you through the steps to becoming a successful makeup artist. Resources and Complements To continue expanding your knowledge and skills in the world of makeup, it is important to explore additional resources and complements. In this chapter, we will recommend books, courses, and workshops that can help you further your education and keep up with the latest trends in the industry. By mastering the art of contouring and highlighting, you will be able to enhance your natural beauty and create stunning makeup looks that will turn heads. So grab your brushes and let's dive into the world of contouring and highlighting!

Facial Corrections: Camouflaging dark circles, blemishes, imperfections, and asymmetries

Facial Corrections: Camouflaging dark circles, blemishes, imperfections, and asymmetries In this chapter, we will focus on one of the most common challenges faced by makeup artists: correcting facial imperfections. Whether it's dark circles under the eyes, blemishes, scars, or asymmetries, knowing how to camouflage these issues is essential for creating flawless makeup looks. Anatomy of the Face: Before we dive into the specifics of correcting facial imperfections, it's important to understand the anatomy of the face. Knowing the different areas of the face and how they interact with each other will help you determine the best approach to correcting any imperfections. Colorimetry: Choosing the correct tones for your skin is crucial when it comes to camouflaging dark circles, blemishes, and other imperfections. Understanding color theory and how different colors interact with each other will allow you to create a seamless and natural-looking finish. Camouflaging Dark Circles: Dark circles under the eyes can be a common issue for many women. To camouflage dark circles, start by applying a color corrector in a shade that counteracts the darkness. Follow up with a concealer that matches your skin tone to blend the color corrector seamlessly. Camouflaging Blemishes and Imperfections: When it comes to blemishes and imperfections, the key is to use a full-coverage concealer that matches your skin tone. Apply the concealer directly to the blemish and gently blend it outwards to create a seamless finish. Set the concealer with a translucent powder to ensure long-lasting coverage. Camouflaging Asymmetries: Asymmetries in the face can be corrected by using makeup to create balance and harmony. Use contouring and highlighting techniques to sculpt the face and create the illusion of symmetry. Remember to blend carefully to avoid harsh lines and create a natural-looking finish. By mastering the art of facial corrections, you will be able to create flawless makeup looks that enhance your natural beauty. Practice these techniques and experiment with different products to find what works best for you. Remember, practice makes perfect, and with dedication and determination, you can become a professional makeup artist capable of transforming any face into a work of art.

Makeup Setting: Techniques to keep your look impeccable all day long

Makeup Setting: Techniques to keep your look impeccable all day long One of the most important aspects of professional makeup application is ensuring that your look stays flawless throughout the day. Whether you're heading to a long day at the office or a special event that lasts into the night, it's crucial to have the right techniques and products in place to keep your makeup looking fresh and beautiful. In this chapter, we will explore some key techniques for setting your makeup to ensure longevity and durability. From primers to setting sprays, we will cover everything you need to know to keep your makeup in place all day long. 1. Primer: Before applying any makeup, it's essential to start with a good primer. This will create a smooth base for your foundation and help your makeup adhere to your skin better. Choose a primer that suits your skin type, whether it's hydrating, mattifying, or pore minimizing. 2. Setting powder: Once you've applied your foundation and concealer, it's important to set everything in place with a setting powder. This will help to prevent your makeup from creasing or sliding off throughout the day. Use a fluffy brush to lightly dust the powder over your face, focusing on areas that tend to get oily. 3. Setting spray: To lock in your makeup and ensure it stays put all day, finish off your look with a setting spray. This will help to seal everything in place and give your makeup a natural, dewy finish. Hold the setting spray a few inches away from your face and spritz evenly over your makeup. 4. Touch-ups: Throughout the day, it's inevitable that your makeup may start to fade or wear off. Keep a few key products in your bag for quick touch-ups, such as a pressed powder, blotting papers, and a lipstick or lip gloss for touch-ups. By following these techniques for setting your makeup, you can ensure that your look stays impeccable all day long. With the right products and tools, you can confidently go about your day knowing that your makeup will stay fresh and beautiful.

Part 3: Makeup for Special Occasions

Makeup for Special Occasions Special occasions call for special makeup looks. Whether you're attending a wedding, a gala, a red carpet event, or any other special event, you want to look your best. In this chapter, we will cover everything you need to know to create stunning makeup looks for any special occasion. 1. Preparing the Skin: Before applying makeup for a special occasion, it's essential to prepare the skin properly. Start by cleansing the face with a gentle cleanser to remove any dirt, oil, and makeup residue. Follow up with a hydrating moisturizer to ensure a smooth and hydrated base for your makeup application. 2. Choosing the Right Foundation: For special occasions, it's important to choose a foundation that not only matches your skin tone but also provides long-lasting coverage. Opt for a full-coverage foundation that will give you a flawless complexion and withstand the test of time. Make sure to blend the foundation seamlessly into your skin, paying special attention to areas that need extra coverage. 3. Eye Makeup: When it comes to eye makeup for special occasions, the possibilities are endless. From smokey eyes to glittery lids, you can get as creative as you want. Consider using eyeshadow colors that complement your outfit and enhance your eye color. Don't forget to apply eyeliner and mascara to define and enhance your eyes. 4. Contouring and Highlighting: Contouring and highlighting are essential steps in creating a sculpted and radiant makeup look for special occasions. Use a contour shade to define your cheekbones, jawline, and nose, and a highlighter to add a luminous glow to your skin. Blend these products seamlessly for a natural and flawless finish. 5. Lip Makeup: Finish off your special occasion makeup look with a stunning lip color. Whether you prefer a classic red lip or a bold berry shade, choose a lipstick that complements your overall look. Make sure to line your lips with a lip liner to prevent feathering and enhance the shape of your lips. 6. Setting the Makeup: To ensure your makeup stays put throughout the event, set it with a setting spray or powder. This will help lock in your makeup and prevent it from fading or creasing. Carry a touch-up kit with you for any necessary touch-ups throughout the day or night. Creating a professional makeup look for special occasions requires practice, patience, and attention to detail. By following the techniques and tips outlined in this chapter, you'll be able to create stunning makeup looks that will make you feel confident and beautiful for any special event.

Daytime Makeup: Natural and sophisticated looks for daytime events

Daytime Makeup: Natural and sophisticated looks for daytime events When it comes to daytime makeup, the key is to enhance your natural beauty while still looking polished and put-together. Whether you're heading to a business meeting, brunch with friends, or a daytime event, it's important to choose makeup that is both sophisticated and appropriate for the occasion. In this chapter, we will explore the techniques and products needed to create natural and sophisticated daytime looks that will leave you feeling confident and beautiful. First and foremost, it's important to start with a clean and moisturized canvas. Proper skincare is essential for achieving a flawless makeup application, so make sure to cleanse, tone, and moisturize your skin before beginning your makeup routine. Next, it's time to choose the right foundation for your skin tone. Color theory plays a crucial role in makeup application, so be sure to choose a foundation that matches your skin perfectly. Use a beauty blender or foundation brush to blend the product seamlessly into your skin, creating a smooth and even base. For daytime events, it's best to opt for a natural eyeshadow look. Stick to neutral shades such as browns, taupes, and soft pinks to enhance your eyes without looking too overdone. Use a fluffy brush to blend the eyeshadow seamlessly into your crease, creating a soft and natural effect. When it comes to eyeliner, a thin line along the upper lash line will help define your eyes without looking too heavy. Use a black or brown eyeliner pencil to create a subtle winged effect, elongating your eyes and adding a touch of sophistication. Finish off your daytime look with a swipe of mascara to lengthen and volumize your lashes. Opt for a waterproof formula to ensure your mascara stays put throughout the day, even in hot and humid weather. For the lips, a nude or pink lipstick will complement your natural makeup look perfectly. Choose a shade that enhances your natural lip color and adds a hint of shine for a polished finish. With the right tools and techniques, you can create natural and sophisticated daytime looks that are perfect for any occasion. Experiment with different products and colors to find what works best for you, and don't be afraid to step out of your comfort zone and try new trends. Remember, makeup is all about enhancing your natural beauty and expressing your unique style. With the tips and tricks outlined in this chapter, you'll be able to create stunning daytime looks that will leave you feeling confident and beautiful all day long.

Evening Makeup: Glamorous and elegant styles for special occasions

Evening Makeup: Glamorous and elegant styles for special occasions When it comes to special occasions, evening makeup is all about creating a glamorous and elegant look that will make you stand out from the crowd. Whether you're attending a formal event, a wedding, or a night out on the town, mastering the art of evening makeup is essential for any professional makeup artist. In this chapter, we will delve into the techniques and tips for creating stunning evening makeup looks that will leave a lasting impression. From dramatic smokey eyes to bold red lips, we will explore a variety of styles and trends that are perfect for any special occasion. Anatomy of the face and colorimetry play a crucial role in evening makeup, as choosing the correct tones for your skin is key to achieving a flawless look. Understanding how to enhance your client's natural features and create a harmonious color palette is essential for creating a stunning evening makeup look. We will cover the application of basic and advanced makeup techniques for eyes, lips, and face, including how to create a flawless base, sculpted cheekbones, and defined brows. From blending eyeshadows to perfecting winged eyeliner, we will walk you through step-by-step instructions on how to achieve a professional evening makeup look. Tricks and tips for creating natural looks, day-to-night transitions, and themed event makeup will also be discussed in this chapter. Whether you're aiming for a soft and romantic look or a bold and dramatic statement, we will provide you with the tools and techniques needed to bring your client's vision to life. Professional makeup techniques such as high definition, contouring, strobing, and 3D makeup will be explored in-depth, giving you the skills and knowledge to elevate your evening makeup looks to the next level. Learn how to create a sculpted face, radiant skin, and luminous highlights that will make your client shine at any special occasion. In addition to technical skills, we will also discuss the ethical, business, and marketing aspects of becoming a successful professional makeup artist. From building your portfolio to networking with clients and industry professionals, we will provide you with the resources and guidance needed to thrive in the competitive world of makeup artistry. By the end of this chapter, you will have the knowledge and confidence to create glamorous and elegant evening makeup looks that will leave a lasting impression on your clients. With the tools and techniques provided in this book, you will be well-equipped to succeed as a professional makeup artist in the exciting and dynamic world of beauty.

Smoky Eye Makeup: Techniques to create an intense and mysterious look

Smoky Eye Makeup Creating a smoky eye look is a classic technique that can instantly add intensity and mystery to your overall makeup. In this chapter, we will explore different techniques to achieve the perfect smoky eye, whether you're going for a soft and subtle look or a bold and dramatic one. 1. Prepping the eyelids: Before diving into creating a smoky eye, it's important to prep your eyelids. Start by applying an eyeshadow primer to ensure your eyeshadow stays in place all day. This will also help the colors pop and blend seamlessly. 2. Choosing the right colors: Traditionally, a smoky eye is created using dark shades such as black, grey, or brown. However, you can also experiment with colors like navy, plum, or even green for a unique twist. The key is to choose shades that complement your eye color and skin tone. 3. Building up the intensity: Start by applying a medium-toned eyeshadow all over your eyelid as a base. Then, use a darker shade to define the crease and outer corner of your eye. Blend the colors seamlessly to create a gradient effect. 4. Adding depth and dimension: To intensify the smoky effect, layer a black or dark brown eyeshadow on the outer corner of your eye and blend it towards the center. This will create a sultry and mysterious look. 5. Enhancing the eyes: To complete the smoky eye look, line your upper and lower lash line with a black eyeliner. You can also add a touch of shimmer on the inner corner of your eyes to make them pop. Finish off with a few coats of mascara for added drama. 6. Tips and tricks: To prevent fallout from dark eyeshadows, do your eye makeup before your foundation. You can also use a piece of tape to create a clean and sharp edge for your eyeshadow. By mastering the art of smoky eye makeup, you can create a versatile look that is perfect for any occasion. Experiment with different colors and techniques to find the smoky eye style that suits you best. Remember, practice makes perfect, so don't be afraid to play around and have fun with your makeup!

Dramatic Eye Makeup: Application of false eyelashes, graphic liners, and vibrant colors

Dramatic Eye Makeup: Application of false eyelashes, graphic liners, and vibrant colors In this chapter, we will explore the exciting world of dramatic eye makeup. From bold false eyelashes to graphic liners and vibrant colors, we will teach you how to create eye-catching looks that will make a statement. False eyelashes are a key component of dramatic eye makeup. They can add volume, length, and drama to your lashes, making your eyes stand out. To apply false eyelashes, start by measuring and trimming them to fit your eye shape. Then, apply a thin layer of eyelash glue to the band of the lashes and wait for it to become tacky before carefully placing them along your natural lash line. Press down gently to secure them in place and blend them with your natural lashes using mascara. Graphic liners are another fun way to add drama to your eye makeup look. Whether you prefer bold winged liner or intricate designs, graphic liners can help you create a unique and eye-catching look. To create a graphic liner look, start by sketching out your desired shape with a pencil liner. Once you are happy with the shape, go over it with a liquid or gel liner for a more precise and long-lasting finish. Vibrant colors are a great way to add a pop of color to your eye makeup look. Whether you prefer bright blues, bold greens, or vibrant purples, experimenting with different colors can help you create a unique and exciting look. To incorporate vibrant colors into your eye makeup, start by applying a neutral base shade to your eyelids. Then, use a small brush to pack on the vibrant color, blending it outwards towards the crease for a seamless finish. By mastering the application of false eyelashes, graphic liners, and vibrant colors, you can create stunning and dramatic eye makeup looks that will turn heads wherever you go. Experiment with different techniques and colors to find what works best for you and don't be afraid to step out of your comfort zone and try something new. Remember, makeup is all about expressing yourself and having fun, so don't be afraid to get creative and experiment with different looks.

Statement Lip Makeup: Red lips, ombre, and special effects

STATEMENT LIP MAKEUP: RED LIPS, OMBRE, AND SPECIAL EFFECTS In this chapter, we will delve into the art of creating statement lip makeup looks that are sure to turn heads. Whether you want to rock a classic red lip, experiment with ombre techniques, or try your hand at special effects makeup, we've got you covered.   Red lips have long been a symbol of glamour and sophistication. To achieve the perfect red lip, start by choosing a shade that complements your skin tone. Fair skin tones can pull off a true red, while medium skin tones look stunning in berry shades. Dark skin tones can rock a deep cherry red with ease. Once you've found the perfect shade, outline your lips with a matching lip liner to prevent feathering and bleeding. Fill in your lips with a lipstick or lip stain, making sure to stay within the lines for a clean finish. For a modern twist on the classic red lip, try a matte or metallic finish for added drama. Ombre lips are a fun and trendy way to play with color and dimension. To create an ombre effect, start by applying a darker shade of lipstick to the outer corners of your lips, blending towards the center. Then, apply a lighter shade to the center of your lips and blend outwards, creating a seamless transition between the two shades. You can also experiment with different color combinations, such as a gradient from red to pink or purple to blue, for a unique and eye-catching look. Special effects lip makeup allows you to unleash your creativity and create one-of-a-kind looks. From glitter lips to holographic finishes, the possibilities are endless. To achieve a glitter lip, start by applying a clear lip gloss to your lips as a base. Then, press a generous amount of glitter onto your lips using a brush or your fingertips. For a holographic effect, layer a holographic lip gloss over a metallic lipstick for a futuristic and ethereal look. Don't be afraid to experiment with different textures and finishes to create a lip look that is truly your own. With the techniques and tips outlined in this chapter, you'll be able to master the art of statement lip makeup and create show-stopping looks that are sure to make a lasting impression. So go ahead, experiment with bold colors, textures, and finishes, and unleash your inner makeup artist. The world is your canvas, so have fun and get creative!

Makeup for Social Events: Weddings, graduations, parties, and celebrations

Makeup for Social Events: Weddings, graduations, parties, and celebrations When it comes to makeup for special events such as weddings, graduations, parties, and celebrations, it's important to create a look that enhances your natural beauty and complements the occasion. In this chapter, we will explore the different techniques and tips to help you achieve the perfect makeup for any social event. For weddings, it's important to consider the theme and style of the event. For a traditional wedding, opt for a classic and timeless look with soft, romantic shades. For a modern wedding, you can experiment with bold colors and trends. When it comes to graduations, parties, and other celebrations, you can have more fun with your makeup and experiment with different styles and looks. One important aspect to consider when doing makeup for social events is the longevity of the makeup. Make sure to use long-lasting products and set your makeup with a setting spray to ensure it stays in place throughout the event. Additionally, consider the lighting of the venue and adjust your makeup accordingly to ensure it looks flawless in photos. For weddings, consider using waterproof products to withstand any tears of joy. For graduations and parties, opt for bold and vibrant colors to make a statement. And for celebrations, experiment with glitter and shimmer to add a touch of glamour to your look. Remember to always start with a well-prepped and moisturized skin to ensure a smooth and flawless application. Use a primer to create a smooth canvas for your makeup and to help it last longer. When it comes to choosing the right foundation and concealer, make sure to match the shade to your skin tone and blend it seamlessly for a natural look. For the eyes, consider using neutral shades for a subtle look or experiment with bold colors for a more dramatic effect. Don't forget to define your brows to frame your face and complete your look. For the lips, choose a color that complements your outfit and overall makeup look. Overall, makeup for social events is all about enhancing your natural beauty and expressing your personal style. Experiment with different techniques and products to find what works best for you and don't be afraid to step out of your comfort zone. With the right tools and techniques, you can create a stunning makeup look for any social event.

Themed Makeup: Carnival, Halloween, costume parties

Themed Makeup: Carnival, Halloween, costume parties Themed makeup is a fun and creative way to express yourself and enhance your look for special events like carnivals, Halloween, and costume parties. In this chapter, we will explore different techniques and ideas to help you stand out and make a statement with your makeup. When it comes to themed makeup, the key is to choose a theme that inspires you and allows you to unleash your creativity. Whether you want to transform into a mystical creature, a glamorous celebrity, or a spooky character, the possibilities are endless. For carnival makeup, think bold and vibrant colors that will make you stand out in the crowd. Experiment with glitter, rhinestones, and bold eye shadows to create a festive and eye-catching look. Don't be afraid to go all out and embrace the spirit of the carnival with your makeup.

Halloween makeup is all about transforming into a character or creature that is spooky, eerie, or downright terrifying. From vampires and witches to zombies and skeletons, the possibilities are endless. Use special effects makeup, prosthetics, and fake blood to create a realistic and frightening look that will impress everyone at the party. Costume parties are a great opportunity to get creative and have fun with your makeup. Whether you want to channel your favorite movie character, historical figure, or mythical creature, the key is to pay attention to the details and bring your character to life with makeup. Use contouring, highlighting, and shading techniques to enhance your features and create a realistic and stunning look. Remember, themed makeup is all about having fun and expressing yourself, so don't be afraid to experiment and try new things. With the techniques and tips in this chapter, you will be able to create show-stopping looks that will wow everyone at your next themed event. So grab your makeup brushes and get ready to unleash your creativity with themed makeup!

Part 4: Advanced Makeup and Special Effects

Advanced Makeup and Special Effects In this chapter, we will delve into the world of advanced makeup techniques and special effects that will take your skills to the next level. Whether you are looking to create a flawless high-definition look or transform yourself into a fantastical creature for a themed event, this chapter has got you covered. Anatomy of the face and colorimetry are essential tools for any makeup artist. Understanding the structure of the face and how different colors interact with each other will help you choose the correct tones for your skin and create a harmonious makeup look. We will explore the application of basic and advanced makeup techniques for eyes, lips, and face. From intricate eye shadow blending to perfecting the art of contouring and highlighting, you will learn how to enhance your features and create stunning looks for any occasion. Tricks and tips for creating natural looks, day, night, and special occasions will be shared in this chapter. Whether you are going for a subtle and understated look or a bold and dramatic one, you will learn how to tailor your makeup to suit the event and your personal style. Professional makeup techniques such as high-definition makeup, contouring, strobing, and 3D makeup will be covered in detail. These techniques are essential for creating flawless looks that will withstand the scrutiny of high-definition cameras and make a statement on the runway or red carpet. Ethical, business, and marketing aspects of being a professional makeup artist will also be discussed in this chapter. From maintaining high standards of hygiene and professionalism to building a successful brand and marketing yourself effectively, you will learn how to navigate the business side of the industry. Lastly, resources and complements to expand your knowledge and continue learning will be provided. Whether you are looking to further your education through workshops and courses or invest in quality tools and products, this chapter will equip you with the information you need to succeed in the competitive world of makeup artistry. By mastering the techniques and concepts covered in this chapter, you will be well on your way to becoming a skilled and successful professional makeup artist. So grab your brushes and get ready to unleash your creativity with the advanced makeup and special effects techniques in this chapter.

High-Definition Makeup: Professional techniques for a flawless finish on camera and events

High-Definition Makeup: Professional techniques for a flawless finish on camera and events In this chapter, we will delve into the world of high-definition makeup, where precision and perfection are key to achieving a flawless finish on camera and for special events. Whether you are a makeup artist looking to enhance your skills or someone who simply wants to master the art of makeup for high-definition settings, this chapter will provide you with the tools and techniques necessary to achieve professional results. Anatomy of the face and colorimetry play a crucial role in high-definition makeup. Understanding the structure of the face and how to choose the correct tones for your skin is essential for creating a seamless look that will translate well on camera. We will explore how to highlight and contour the face to create dimension and enhance your natural features. We will also cover the application of basic and advanced makeup techniques for eyes, lips, and face. From creating the perfect winged eyeliner to achieving a flawless base, you will learn how to master the techniques that will elevate your makeup game to the next level. Tricks and tips for creating natural looks, day-to-night transitions, and special occasion makeup will also be discussed. Whether you are looking to create a soft and subtle look for a daytime event or a bold and glamorous look for a night out, you will learn how to tailor your makeup to suit any occasion. Professional makeup techniques such as contouring, strobing, and 3D makeup will be covered in detail. These techniques are crucial for achieving a flawless finish on camera and for creating a three-dimensional look that will make your features pop. Lastly, we will touch on the ethical, business, and marketing aspects of becoming a successful professional makeup artist. From building your portfolio to networking with clients, you will learn how to take your passion for makeup and turn it into a successful career. In conclusion, this chapter will provide you with the knowledge and skills necessary to master high-definition makeup techniques and elevate your makeup game to a professional level. By following the step-by-step guidance provided in this chapter, you will be able to achieve a flawless finish on camera and for special events, ensuring that you always look your best.

Advanced Contouring: Extreme facial definition, sculpted cheekbones, and profiled noses

Advanced Contouring: Extreme facial definition, sculpted cheekbones, and profiled noses In this chapter, we will delve deep into the world of advanced contouring techniques to achieve extreme facial definition, sculpted cheekbones, and profiled noses. Contouring is a powerful tool that can completely transform the shape and structure of the face, creating a more defined and sculpted look. The key to successful contouring is understanding the anatomy of the face and colorimetry to choose the correct tones for your skin. By using a combination of dark and light shades, you can create the illusion of shadow and light to enhance your features and create a more symmetrical and balanced look. To begin, start by applying a matte bronzer or contour powder to the hollows of the cheeks, temples, jawline, and sides of the nose. Blend well to ensure a seamless and natural finish. Next, apply a highlighter to the high points of the face, such as the cheekbones, brow bone, and the bridge of the nose, to add dimension and luminosity. For sculpted cheekbones, use a contour shade slightly darker than your skin tone to create a shadow underneath the cheekbones. Blend upwards towards the temples for a lifted effect. Then, apply a highlighter to the tops of the cheekbones to accentuate their shape and create a radiant glow. To profile the nose, use a contour shade to create shadows on the sides of the nose to make it appear slimmer and more defined. Apply a highlighter down the bridge of the nose to draw attention to this area and create the illusion of a straighter and more sculpted nose. Remember to blend well and use a light hand when applying contour and highlight shades to avoid a harsh and unnatural look. Practice makes perfect, so don't be afraid to experiment and try different techniques to find what works best for your unique face shape. By mastering advanced contouring techniques, you can enhance your natural beauty and create a flawless and sculpted look that will turn heads wherever you go. With practice and patience, you can become a master of contouring and create stunning makeup looks that will leave a lasting impression.

Strobing: Strategic highlighting for a radiant and vibrant look

Strobing: Strategic highlighting for a radiant and vibrant look Strobing is a makeup technique that focuses on strategically highlighting certain areas of the face to create a radiant and vibrant look. This technique is all about enhancing the natural glow of the skin, rather than contouring and sculpting the face. To achieve the perfect strobing effect, it's important to select the right highlighter for your skin tone. Choose a highlighter that complements your skin tone and has a shimmering finish to create a luminous effect. Apply the highlighter to the high points of your face, such as the cheekbones, brow bones, bridge of the nose, and cupid's bow. When applying highlighter, use a light hand and build up the product gradually to avoid a harsh and overly shimmery look. Blend the highlighter seamlessly into your skin using a fluffy brush or a damp makeup sponge for a more natural finish. Strobing is a versatile technique that can be customized to suit different makeup looks. For a subtle and natural look, opt for a cream or liquid highlighter and apply it sparingly for a soft glow. For a more intense and glamorous look, choose a powder highlighter with a high shimmer finish and layer it for a more dramatic effect. Experiment with different shades and finishes of highlighters to find the perfect one for your skin tone and desired look. Remember that strobing is all about enhancing your natural beauty and creating a radiant and luminous complexion. In this chapter, we will explore the art of strobing in detail, from choosing the right highlighter to applying it strategically for a flawless finish. With the techniques and tips provided in this book, you'll be able to master the art of strobing and achieve a radiant and vibrant look every time.

3D Makeup: Creating volume and dimension on the face using advanced techniques

3D Makeup: Creating volume and dimension on the face using advanced techniques In this chapter, we will delve into the world of 3D makeup, a technique that allows you to create depth and dimension on the face using advanced techniques. By mastering 3D makeup, you will be able to enhance your features and create a flawless, sculpted look that will turn heads wherever you go. To begin, let's start by understanding the anatomy of the face and how color theory plays a crucial role in choosing the correct tones for your skin. By understanding the natural shadows and highlights of the face, you will be able to strategically place makeup to enhance your features and create a three-dimensional effect. Next, we will explore the application of basic and advanced makeup techniques for eyes, lips, and face. From creating a flawless base using foundation and concealer to sculpting the cheeks with contour and highlight, you will learn how to achieve a professional finish that is sure to impress. Tricks and tips for creating natural looks, day-to-night makeup, and special occasion makeup will also be covered in this chapter. Whether you're looking to enhance your everyday look or create a show-stopping makeup look for a special event, you will learn the techniques needed to achieve stunning results. Moving on to the main focus of this chapter, we will delve into professional makeup techniques for high definition, contouring, strobing, and 3D makeup. By mastering these advanced techniques, you will be able to create a sculpted, three-dimensional look that will enhance your natural beauty and make you stand out from the crowd. Finally, we will touch on the ethical, business, and marketing aspects of becoming a successful professional makeup artist. By understanding the importance of professionalism, ethics, and marketing yourself effectively, you will be able to build a successful career in the competitive world of makeup artistry. In conclusion, this chapter will equip you with the knowledge and skills needed to master the art of 3D makeup and create stunning, three-dimensional looks that will leave a lasting impression. By following the step-by-step instructions and practicing the techniques outlined in this chapter, you will be well on your way to becoming a professional makeup artist with a flair for creating volume and dimension on the face.

Artistic Makeup: Character design, special effects, and creative transformations

Artistic Makeup: Character design, special effects, and creative transformations Artistic makeup goes beyond the traditional beauty looks and allows you to unleash your creativity and imagination. In this chapter, we will explore the exciting world of character design, special effects, and creative transformations through makeup. Character Design: Creating a character through makeup involves understanding the personality, backstory, and characteristics of the individual you are transforming. Whether it's a fantasy creature, historical figure, or a fictional character, the key is to bring them to life through makeup. This requires careful planning, attention to detail, and a keen eye for design. Special Effects: Special effects makeup involves the use of prosthetics, latex, and other materials to create realistic wounds, scars, aging effects, and more. This technique is commonly used in film, theater, and television to enhance the storytelling and create believable characters. Learning how to sculpt, mold, and apply special effects makeup will take your skills to the next level. Creative Transformations: Creative transformations allow you to push the boundaries of makeup and experiment with unconventional looks. Whether it's avant-garde fashion, editorial makeup, or abstract art, the goal is to challenge the norms and create visually stunning designs. This is where you can truly express yourself and showcase your unique style as a makeup artist. In this chapter, you will learn: - Techniques for character design, including prosthetic application, aging effects, and fantasy makeup. - Special effects makeup tricks, such as creating wounds, bruises, and realistic textures. - Tips for creative transformations, including using unconventional materials, colors, and shapes. - How to incorporate storytelling and emotion into your makeup designs. - Professional resources for sourcing materials, inspiration, and continuing education in artistic makeup. By mastering the art of artistic makeup, you will open up a world of possibilities and opportunities in the makeup industry. Whether you aspire to work in film, theater, fashion, or special events, the skills you learn in this chapter will set you apart as a versatile and innovative makeup artist. Let your creativity soar and transform the ordinary into the extraordinary with artistic makeup.

Makeup for Mature Skin: Tips and techniques to enhance beauty at all ages

Makeup for Mature Skin: Tips and techniques to enhance beauty at all ages As we age, our skin changes and so does our makeup routine. In this chapter, we will explore the best tips and techniques to enhance the beauty of mature skin. 1. Skincare for mature skin: Before applying makeup, it is essential to have a good skincare routine. Mature skin tends to be drier and more delicate, so it is important to use hydrating and nourishing products. Make sure to cleanse, tone, and moisturize your skin before starting your makeup routine. 2. Color theory for mature skin: As we age, our skin tone may change, and it is important to choose the right colors for your makeup. Stick to warmer tones for a more youthful look, and avoid harsh colors that can make you look older. Neutral shades are always a safe bet for mature skin. 3. Foundation and concealer: When applying foundation and concealer on mature skin, opt for a lightweight formula that won't settle into fine lines and wrinkles. Use a beauty sponge or brush to blend the product seamlessly into the skin, creating a flawless finish. Concealer can be used to cover dark circles and age spots, but be careful not to apply too much product, as it can accentuate fine lines. 4. Eye makeup for mature skin: For mature eyes, it is best to stick to neutral shades and avoid shimmery or glittery eyeshadows that can draw attention to fine lines. Use matte eyeshadows to create a subtle and sophisticated look. Don't forget to curl your lashes and apply mascara to open up the eyes. 5. Lip makeup for mature skin: Choose creamy and hydrating lipsticks in soft, natural shades to enhance the lips. Avoid dark lip colors that can make your lips look smaller. Lip liners can help define the lips and prevent lipstick from bleeding into fine lines. 6. Blush and contouring: Blush can add a youthful flush to the cheeks, but be careful not to apply too much product. Use a light hand and blend the blush well into the skin for a natural look. Contouring can help define the features of the face, but keep it subtle and avoid harsh lines. 7. Setting spray and finishing touches: To ensure your makeup lasts all day, use a setting spray to lock in your look. Finish off with a dusting of translucent powder to set your makeup and reduce shine. By following these tips and techniques, you can enhance the beauty of mature skin and create a radiant and youthful look at any age. Remember, makeup is meant to enhance your natural beauty, so embrace your age and feel confident in your skin.

Makeup for Different Ethnicities: Considerations and tips for adapting makeup to every skin tone

Makeup for Different Ethnicities When it comes to

makeup, one size does not fit all. Different ethnicities have unique skin tones and features that require special considerations when it comes to choosing and applying makeup. In this chapter, we will discuss some tips and guidelines for adapting makeup to every skin tone. 1. Understanding Skin Tones Before we dive into specific tips for different ethnicities, it's important to understand the basics of skin tones. Skin tones can be classified into warm, cool, or neutral undertones. Warm undertones have a yellow or golden hue, while cool undertones have a pink or blue hue. Neutral undertones have a mix of both warm and cool tones. When choosing makeup for different ethnicities, it's essential to consider the undertones of the skin. For example, individuals with warmer undertones may look best in makeup with golden or bronze tones, while those with cooler undertones may prefer makeup with pink or blue undertones. 2. Makeup Tips for Different Ethnicities a. Asian Skin Tones: Asian skin tones often have yellow undertones. When applying makeup to Asian skin, opt for foundations and concealers with yellow or golden undertones to match the skin perfectly. Avoid using shades that are too light or too dark, as they can look unnatural on Asian skin. b. Black/African-American Skin Tones: Black/African-American skin tones can vary widely, from deep ebony to rich chocolate. When selecting makeup for darker skin tones, choose foundations and concealers that match the skin tone closely. Avoid shades that are too light or ashy, as they can make the skin appear dull. c. Hispanic/Latina Skin Tones: Hispanic/Latina skin tones often have warm undertones with a mix of olive and golden hues. When applying makeup to Hispanic/Latina skin, choose warm-toned foundations and blushes to complement the skin tone. Avoid shades that are too cool or ashy, as they can clash with the warm undertones. d. Middle Eastern Skin Tones: Middle Eastern skin tones can range from fair to olive to deep tan. When choosing makeup for Middle Eastern skin, opt for foundations and concealers with warm undertones to enhance the natural beauty of the skin. Avoid shades that are too light or too dark, as they can look unnatural on Middle Eastern skin. Remember, these are just general guidelines, and it's essential to consider individual skin tones and features when applying makeup. Experiment with different shades and products to find what works best for each ethnicity. In conclusion, adapting makeup to different ethnicities requires an understanding of skin tones and features. By following these tips and guidelines, you can create stunning makeup looks that enhance the natural beauty of every ethnicity. Experiment, practice, and have fun exploring the world of makeup for different skin tones.

Part 5: Professional Makeup Aspects

Part 5: Professional Makeup Aspects In this section, we will delve into the various aspects of professional makeup that will help you become a successful makeup artist. From understanding the anatomy of the face to mastering color theory, this chapter will provide you with the knowledge and skills you need to excel in the world of makeup. Anatomy of the face is crucial for any makeup artist. Understanding the different parts of the face, such as the eyes, lips, and cheeks, will help you create looks that enhance your client's natural beauty. By knowing how to highlight and contour each feature, you can create a flawless finish that will leave your clients feeling confident and beautiful. Colorimetry is another important aspect of professional makeup. Choosing the right tones for your client's skin can make all the difference in how their makeup looks. By understanding color theory and how different shades interact with each other, you can create a harmonious and flattering look that complements your client's complexion. In this chapter, we will also cover the application of basic and advanced makeup techniques for the eyes, lips, and face. From creating a natural look for everyday wear to a glamorous look for a special occasion, you will learn how to use different techniques and products to achieve the desired effect. Tricks and tips for creating different makeup looks will also be discussed in this section. Whether you are looking to create a natural look, a smoky eye for a night out, or a bold look for a themed event, this chapter will provide you with the tools and techniques you need to bring your vision to life. Professional makeup techniques such as high definition, contouring, strobing, and 3D makeup will also be covered in this chapter. These advanced techniques can take your makeup skills to the next level, allowing you to create looks that are flawless and camera-ready. Finally, we will discuss the ethical, business, and marketing aspects of becoming a successful professional makeup artist. From building your portfolio to networking with clients and industry professionals, this chapter will provide you with the tools and resources you need to succeed in the competitive world of makeup artistry. By mastering the techniques and skills covered in this chapter, you will be well on your way to becoming a successful and sought-after professional makeup artist. With dedication, practice, and a passion for makeup, you can turn your love for beauty into a rewarding and fulfilling career.

Hygiene and Sanitization: Essential practices for a professional and safe work environment

Hygiene and Sanitization: Essential practices for a professional and safe work environment Ensuring proper hygiene and sanitization practices is crucial in the world of professional makeup. As a makeup artist, it is your responsibility to provide a safe and clean environment for your clients. Not only does this protect the health and well-being of your clients, but it also reflects your professionalism and dedication to your craft. Here are some essential practices to follow when it comes to hygiene and sanitization: 1. Clean and sanitize your tools: It is important to regularly clean and sanitize your makeup brushes, sponges, and other tools. Use a gentle brush cleanser or a mixture of water and gentle soap to clean your brushes after each use. You can also use alcohol or a specialized brush sanitizer to disinfect your tools. 2. Wash your hands: Before starting any makeup application, make sure to wash your hands thoroughly with soap and water. This will help prevent the spread of germs and bacteria. 3. Use disposable tools: Whenever possible, use disposable tools such as mascara wands, lip brushes, and disposable sponges. This will help prevent cross-contamination and ensure a safe and hygienic environment for your clients. 4. Sanitize your makeup products: Regularly sanitize your makeup products, especially those that come in direct contact with the skin, such as lipsticks and eyeliners. You can use alcohol or specialized makeup sanitizing sprays to disinfect your products. 5. Maintain a clean workspace: Keep your makeup station clean and organized at all times. Wipe down surfaces with disinfectant wipes before and after each client to prevent the spread of germs and bacteria. By following these hygiene and sanitization practices, you can create a professional and safe work environment for both yourself and your clients. Remember, cleanliness is key to success in the world of professional makeup.

Ethics and Professionalism: Values and fundamental principles in the makeup industry

Ethics and Professionalism: Values and fundamental

principles in the makeup industry In the world of makeup artistry, it is crucial to uphold the highest ethical standards and professionalism. As a professional makeup artist, you are not only responsible for enhancing the natural beauty of your clients, but also for ensuring their well-being and satisfaction.   One of the fundamental principles in the makeup industry is respect for diversity and individuality. Every client is unique, with their own preferences, skin tones, and features. It is important to always listen to your clients' needs and desires, and to work together to create a look that complements their personal style. Another key value in the makeup industry is integrity. As a makeup artist, you have the power to transform someone's appearance and boost their confidence. It is essential to always be honest with your clients about the products you are using, the techniques you are applying, and the expected results. Professionalism is also crucial in the makeup industry. This means arriving on time for appointments, maintaining a clean and organized workspace, and always presenting yourself in a polished and professional manner. Building strong relationships with your clients based on trust and reliability is essential for a successful career in makeup artistry. In addition to ethical and professional values, it is important for makeup artists to stay informed about the latest trends, techniques, and products in the industry. Continuing education and training are key to staying competitive and offering the best services to your clients. By upholding these values and fundamental principles in the makeup industry, you will not only build a strong reputation as a professional makeup artist, but also create lasting relationships with your clients based on trust, respect, and integrity.

Marketing and Personal Promotion: Creating a personal brand and strategies to attract clients

Marketing and Personal Promotion Creating a personal brand and strategies to attract clients In the competitive world of professional makeup, it is essential to not only have the skills and techniques necessary to excel, but also to effectively market yourself and create a personal brand that will attract clients. In this chapter, we will delve into the key strategies to help you establish your presence in the industry and grow your client base. 1. Define Your Unique Selling Proposition (USP) Before you can effectively market yourself, you must first identify what sets you apart from other makeup artists. What makes your services unique? Do you specialize in a certain type of makeup application, such as bridal or special effects? Do you have a signature style that clients love? By defining your USP, you can better target your marketing efforts and attract clients who are looking for what you have to offer. 2. Build Your Online Presence In today's digital age, having a strong online presence is crucial for attracting clients. Create a professional website that showcases your work, services, and pricing. Utilize social media platforms such as Instagram,

Facebook, and LinkedIn to share your portfolio, engage with potential clients, and build your brand. Consider creating a blog or YouTube channel to share makeup tutorials, beauty tips, and behind-the-scenes content to further establish yourself as an expert in the field. 3. Network and Collaborate Networking is a powerful tool for expanding your client base and building relationships within the industry. Attend makeup trade shows, beauty expos, and industry events to connect with other professionals and potential clients. Collaborate with photographers, models, and hair stylists on photo shoots and projects to showcase your skills and expand your portfolio. By building a strong network of contacts, you can increase your visibility and attract new clients through referrals and word-of-mouth. 4. Offer Special Promotions and Packages To attract new clients and retain existing ones, consider offering special promotions and packages. For example, you could offer discounted rates for bridal parties, makeup lessons, or group bookings. Create loyalty programs or referral incentives to encourage repeat business and client referrals. By providing value-added services and incentives, you can differentiate yourself from the competition and attract clients who are looking for a professional makeup artist who goes above and beyond. 5. Seek Feedback and Reviews Feedback and reviews are essential for building credibility and attracting new clients. Encourage your clients to leave reviews on your website, social media pages, and online review platforms such as Yelp and Google My Business. Actively seek feedback from clients to improve your services and address any issues or concerns. By showcasing positive reviews and testimonials, you can build trust with potential clients and demonstrate your expertise and professionalism. By implementing these strategies and creating a strong personal brand, you can effectively market yourself as a professional makeup artist and attract clients who are looking for your unique skills and services. Remember to stay true to your brand, consistently deliver exceptional service, and continue to grow and evolve as a makeup artist to stand out in the competitive industry.

Business Management: Organization, administration, and customer service in a makeup studio

Business Management: Organization, administration, and customer service in a makeup studio In order to run a successful makeup studio, it is essential to have a strong foundation in business management. This includes organization, administration, and top-notch customer service. In this chapter, we will delve into the key aspects of running a makeup studio and how to ensure that your business thrives. Organization is key when it comes to running a makeup studio. You need to have a system in place for scheduling appointments, managing inventory, and keeping track of your finances. This includes creating a calendar to schedule client appointments, keeping track of your supplies and making sure you have enough on hand, and keeping detailed records of your income and expenses. Administration is another crucial aspect of running a makeup studio. This includes keeping your studio clean and organized, managing your time effectively, and staying on top of your paperwork. You also need to have a system in place for ordering supplies, managing your social media accounts, and keeping in touch with your clients. Customer service is perhaps the most important aspect of running a makeup studio. Your clients are the lifeblood of your business, so it is essential to treat them with the utmost care and respect. This includes being friendly and welcoming, listening to their needs and concerns, and going above and beyond to exceed their expectations. It also means being professional and reliable, always showing up on time and delivering high-quality services. By focusing on organization, administration, and customer service, you can ensure that your makeup studio runs smoothly and successfully. This will not only help you attract and retain clients, but also build a strong reputation in the industry. Remember, running a makeup studio is not just about applying makeup – it is about creating a positive and memorable experience for your clients.

Makeup Trends: Analysis of the latest trends and their professional application

Makeup Trends: Analysis of the latest trends and their

professional application In the ever-evolving world of makeup, it is crucial for professional makeup artists to stay up-to-date with the latest trends. This chapter will provide an in-depth analysis of the current makeup trends and how to effectively apply them in a professional setting. One of the key trends that has been dominating the makeup scene is the focus on natural and glowing skin. The 'no makeup' makeup look has become increasingly popular, with an emphasis on using lightweight products to enhance the skin's natural beauty. Professional makeup artists must master the art of creating flawless skin by using techniques such as color correction, foundation matching, and strategic highlighting and contouring. Another trend that has been making waves in the beauty industry is the resurgence of bold and colorful eyeshadow looks. From bright neon hues to shimmering metallics, there are endless possibilities when it comes to creating eye-catching eye makeup looks. Professional makeup artists should experiment with different color combinations and techniques to stay ahead of the curve. In addition to vibrant eyeshadow looks, statement lips have also been a major trend in recent years. Bold reds, deep berries, and even unconventional shades like blues and greens have been gracing the runways and red carpets. Professional makeup artists must have a keen eye for color theory and be able to recommend the perfect lip color to complement their client's overall look. Contouring, strobing, and 3D makeup techniques have also been popular trends that can elevate any makeup look.

Professional makeup artists should be well-versed in these techniques, as they can help enhance facial features and create a more sculpted appearance. Overall, staying on top of the latest makeup trends is essential for professional makeup artists looking to excel in their careers. By mastering the art of applying these trends in a professional setting, makeup artists can showcase their skills and creativity, ultimately setting themselves apart in the competitive beauty industry.

Runway and Editorial Makeup: Techniques and styles for the fashion world

Runway and Editorial Makeup: Techniques and styles for the fashion world In the fast-paced and ever-evolving world of fashion, makeup plays a crucial role in creating the perfect look to complement the designer's vision. From high fashion runways to editorial shoots in magazines, the makeup artist must be skilled in a variety of techniques and styles to bring the designer's creations to life. In this chapter, we will explore the key techniques and styles used in runway and editorial makeup, as well as tips and tricks to help you succeed in this competitive industry. 1. Runway Makeup Techniques: Runway makeup is all about making a statement. Bold colors, graphic shapes, and avant-garde designs are often seen on the catwalk. To achieve the perfect runway look, it is essential to have a strong understanding of color theory and the ability to create flawless skin. Techniques such as contouring, highlighting, and sculpting can help enhance facial features and create a striking look that will stand out on the runway. 2. Editorial Makeup Styles: Editorial makeup is all about creativity and pushing boundaries. From high fashion editorials to beauty spreads in magazines, editorial makeup allows the artist to experiment with different styles and techniques. Whether it's creating a natural, dewy look for a beach shoot or a dramatic, smokey eye for a high fashion editorial, the key is to adapt to the photographer's vision and bring it to life through makeup. 3. Tips for Success in the Fashion World: To succeed in the competitive world of fashion makeup, it is essential to stay current with the latest trends and techniques. Networking with photographers, designers, and models can help you build connections and secure opportunities in the industry. Additionally, having a strong portfolio that showcases your skills and creativity is crucial for attracting clients and landing jobs in the fashion world. 4. Resources and Further Learning: As a professional makeup artist, it is important to continue learning and expanding your skills. Attending workshops, taking courses, and keeping up to date with industry trends can help you stay ahead of the competition and excel in your career. There are many resources available, both online and offline, to help you further your knowledge and grow as a makeup artist. In conclusion, runway and editorial makeup require a high level of skill, creativity, and adaptability. By mastering the techniques and styles outlined in this chapter, you will be well-equipped to succeed in the fast-paced and exciting world of fashion makeup. Remember to stay inspired, continue learning, and never stop pushing the boundaries of your creativity.

Film and Television Makeup: Characterization and demands of the audiovisual medium

Film and Television Makeup: Characterization and demands of the audiovisual medium In the world of film and television, makeup plays a crucial role in creating characters and bringing stories to life. Whether you're working on a period drama, a sci-fi epic, or a romantic comedy, mastering the art of characterization through makeup is essential for any professional makeup artist. Understanding the demands of the audiovisual medium is key to creating makeup looks that not only look good in person but also translate well on camera. The camera can be unforgiving, picking up every detail and flaw, so it's important to use techniques that will enhance the features of the actors and actresses while still staying true to the character they're portraying. When it comes to film and television makeup, attention to detail is paramount. From creating subtle, natural looks for everyday scenes to bold, dramatic looks for special effects, a makeup artist must be able to adapt to the specific requirements of each project. This may involve working with prosthetics, wigs, and special effects makeup to transform actors into their characters. Color theory also plays a crucial role in film and television makeup. Understanding how different colors interact with each other and how they appear on camera is essential for creating looks that will stand out on screen. Additionally, knowledge of lighting techniques and how they affect makeup application is key to ensuring that the makeup looks flawless in any lighting condition. In this chapter, we will explore the various techniques and tricks used by professional makeup artists in the film and television industry. From creating aging makeup to enhancing facial features for high-definition cameras, you will learn how to master the art of characterization through makeup. We will also discuss the ethical, business, and marketing aspects of working in the film and television industry, as well as provide resources and recommendations for further expanding your knowledge in this exciting field. By the end of this chapter, you will have the skills and confidence to tackle any makeup challenge that comes your way in the world of film and television. Whether you're creating a glamorous red carpet look or a terrifying monster makeup, this chapter will equip you with the tools and techniques necessary to excel in this demanding yet rewarding industry.

Special Effects Makeup: Creating prosthetics, wounds, and realistic transformations

Special Effects Makeup: Creating prosthetics, wounds, and realistic transformations Special effects makeup is a fascinating and essential skill for any professional makeup artist. In this chapter, we will delve into the world of creating prosthetics, wounds, and realistic transformations using makeup techniques that will elevate your artistry to the next level. Creating Prosthetics: Prosthetics are a crucial element in special effects makeup, allowing you to transform a person's appearance dramatically. To create prosthetics, you will need to have a good understanding of anatomy and sculpting techniques. Start by studying the anatomy of the face and practicing sculpting with clay or wax to create realistic prosthetic pieces. Once you have your prosthetic piece sculpted, you will need to cast it in a material such as silicone or gelatin to create a flexible and lifelike appliance. Make sure to blend the edges of the prosthetic seamlessly into the skin using adhesive and makeup to create a seamless transition. Creating Wounds: Wounds are another essential element in special effects makeup, adding realism and drama to your creations. To create wounds, you can use a variety of materials such as latex, wax, and gelatin to achieve different effects. Experiment with different textures and colors to create realistic looking wounds, bruises, and cuts. To make wounds look even more realistic, use makeup techniques such as shading, highlighting, and blood effects to add depth and dimension. Remember to consider the anatomy of the face when creating wounds to ensure they look realistic and believable. Realistic

Transformations: Realistic transformations are the ultimate goal of special effects makeup, allowing you to completely change a person's appearance. Whether you want to age someone, turn them into a creature, or create a fantasy character, the possibilities are endless with special effects makeup. To achieve realistic transformations, you will need to master advanced makeup techniques such as contouring, highlighting, and shading to create dimension and depth. Experiment with different colors, textures, and techniques to bring your transformations to life. In conclusion, special effects makeup is a versatile and exciting skill that allows you to create prosthetics, wounds, and realistic transformations. By mastering these techniques, you will be able to take your artistry to the next level and create truly unforgettable looks. Experiment, practice, and have fun exploring the world of special effects makeup!

Part 6: Resources and Supplements

Resources and Supplements In order to truly excel in the world of professional makeup, it is essential to have access to a variety of resources and supplements that can help expand your knowledge and skills. In this chapter, we will explore some of the best resources available to makeup artists, as well as supplements that can further enhance your expertise. One of the most valuable resources for makeup artists is the internet. There are countless websites, blogs, and online courses that can provide valuable information and tutorials on everything from basic makeup techniques to advanced contouring and strobing. Some popular websites for makeup artists include Makeup Artist Magazine, Beautylish, and Makeup Geek. Another valuable resource for makeup artists is books. There are a plethora of makeup books available that cover a wide range of topics, from color theory to special effects makeup. Some must-have books for makeup artists include "Making Faces" by Kevyn Aucoin, "Bobbi Brown Makeup Manual" by Bobbi Brown, and "Face Forward" by Kevyn Aucoin. Supplements such as workshops, seminars, and masterclasses can also be incredibly beneficial for makeup artists looking to expand their skills. These events provide hands-on experience and the opportunity to learn from industry professionals. Some popular makeup workshops and seminars include The Makeup Show, IMATS (International Makeup Artist Trade Show), and Mastered. In addition to these resources, it is important for makeup artists to stay up to date on the latest trends and techniques in the industry. Subscribing to industry magazines such as Makeup Artist Magazine and attending trade shows and conventions can help you stay informed and inspired. By utilizing these resources and supplements, you can continue to grow and evolve as a professional makeup artist, mastering new techniques and staying ahead of the curve in this ever-changing industry.

Glossary of Terms: Definitions of key words and relevant concepts in the world of makeup

Glossary of Terms In the world of makeup, there are many terms and concepts that may be unfamiliar to beginners. This glossary will help you understand key words and relevant concepts to become a professional makeup artist. 1. Primer: A product applied before makeup to create a smooth canvas and help makeup last longer. 2. Foundation: A base makeup product that evens out skin tone and provides a base for other makeup. 3. Concealer: A product used to cover imperfections such as dark circles, blemishes, and discoloration. 4. Contouring: Using makeup to define and enhance the natural contours of the face, such as cheekbones, jawline, and nose. 5. Strobing: A technique that involves highlighting areas of the face to create a dewy, luminous glow. 6. Setting powder: A powder used to set makeup and reduce shine. 7. Eyeshadow: Pigmented powder or cream used to add color to the eyelids. 8. Eyeliner: A product used to define the eyes and create different looks, such as winged liner or smoky eyes. 9. Mascara: A product used to enhance and darken the eyelashes. 10. Lipstick: A product used to add color to the lips. 11. Lip liner: A product used to define the lips and prevent lipstick from bleeding. 12. Blush: A product used to add color to the cheeks and create a healthy, flushed look. 13. Highlighter: A product used to add a subtle glow to the high points of the face. 14. Makeup brushes: Tools used to apply makeup products to the face and eyes. 15. Color theory: The study of how colors interact and complement each other in makeup application. By familiarizing yourself with these terms and concepts, you will be better equipped to navigate the world of makeup and become a professional artist. Practice using these techniques and products to hone your skills and create stunning looks for yourself and others.

Recommended Products and Brands: Guide to selecting high-quality makeup products

Recommended Products and Brands: Guide to selecting high-quality makeup products When it comes to makeup, using high-quality products can make a world of difference in the final result. In this chapter, we will explore some of the top recommended brands and products that professional makeup artists swear by. 1. Foundation: - Make Up For Ever Ultra HD Foundation: This foundation provides a flawless, natural finish that looks great on camera and in person. - NARS Sheer Glow Foundation: Known for its buildable coverage and luminous finish, this foundation is perfect for creating a radiant complexion. - MAC Studio Fix Fluid Foundation: A cult favorite among makeup artists, this foundation offers long-lasting coverage with a matte finish. 2. Concealer: - Tarte Shape Tape Concealer: This full-coverage concealer is perfect for concealing dark circles, blemishes, and imperfections. - Urban Decay Naked Skin Concealer: With its lightweight formula and buildable coverage, this concealer is great for brightening the under-eye area. - Maybelline Instant Age Rewind Concealer: An affordable option that still delivers great coverage and brightening effects. 3. Eyeshadow: - Anastasia Beverly Hills Modern Renaissance Palette: This palette features a range of highly pigmented shades that blend seamlessly for endless eye looks. - Morphe 350 Nature Glow Eyeshadow Palette: A favorite among makeup artists for its mix of matte and shimmer shades, perfect for creating both natural and bold looks. - ColourPop Super Shock Eyeshadows: These creamy eyeshadows come in a variety of colors and finishes, making them versatile for any makeup look. 4. Lipstick: - MAC Lipsticks: Known for their wide range of shades and finishes, MAC lipsticks are a staple in any makeup artist's kit. - Fenty Beauty Mattemoiselle Plush Matte Lipstick: These lipsticks offer intense color payoff with a comfortable, long-wearing formula. - NYX Soft Matte Lip Cream: Affordable and available in a wide range of shades, these lip creams are perfect for creating a matte lip look. 5. Setting Spray: - Urban Decay All Nighter Setting Spray: This setting spray locks makeup in place for up to 16 hours, ensuring your look stays flawless all day and night. - MAC Fix+: A hydrating mist that can be used before or after makeup application to refresh the skin and set makeup. - Morphe Continuous Setting Mist: This fine mist setting spray helps to keep makeup in place while giving the skin a natural, dewy finish. By investing in high-quality makeup products from reputable brands, you can achieve professional-looking results that last. Experiment with different products to find what works best for you and your clients, and don't be afraid to mix and match to create unique makeup looks. Remember, the key to great makeup is not only in the application technique but also in the products you use.

Inspiration and References: Artists, trends, and styles to broaden your creativity

Inspiration and References As a professional makeup artist, it is important to constantly seek inspiration and stay up-to-date with the latest trends and styles in the industry. Drawing inspiration from artists, trends, and styles can help broaden your creativity and push you to think outside the box when it comes to creating makeup looks. One of the best ways to stay inspired is by following and studying the work of renowned makeup artists. Take note of their techniques, color choices, and overall aesthetic to see how you can incorporate some of their signature styles into your own work. Some artists that you may find inspiring include Pat McGrath, Lisa Eldridge, and Charlotte Tilbury. In addition to following individual artists, keeping up with current trends in the makeup industry is essential. Whether it's the latest runway looks, red carpet glam, or social media makeup trends, staying informed about what's popular can help you stay relevant and adaptable in your work. Experimenting with different styles and techniques is also key to expanding your creativity as a makeup artist. Try recreating looks from different eras, cultures, or even fictional characters to challenge yourself and push your skills to the next level. Lastly, don't be afraid to look outside of the makeup world for inspiration. Fashion, art, nature, and even architecture can all serve as sources of inspiration for creating unique and innovative makeup looks. By immersing yourself in the work of other artists, staying current with trends, and exploring different styles and references, you can continue to grow and evolve as a professional makeup artist. Remember, the possibilities are endless when it comes to makeup, so don't be afraid to think outside the box and let your creativity shine.

Online Resources: Tutorials, blogs, and learning platforms to keep improving

Online Resources: Tutorials, blogs, and learning platforms to keep improving In today's digital age, there are countless resources available online to help you continue improving and honing your makeup skills. Whether you're a beginner looking to learn the basics or a seasoned professional wanting to stay up-to-date on the latest trends and techniques, the internet is a treasure trove of information waiting to be explored. Tutorials: One of the best ways to learn new makeup techniques is by watching tutorials. Platforms like YouTube, Instagram, and TikTok are filled with talented makeup artists who share their skills and knowledge through step-by-step videos. Whether you want to master a smokey eye, perfect your contouring skills, or learn how to create a flawless base, there is a tutorial out there for you. Blogs: Makeup blogs are another great resource for staying informed and inspired. Many beauty bloggers share product reviews, makeup tips, and tutorials on their websites. They often provide in-depth explanations of techniques and product recommendations, making them a valuable source of information for both beginners and experts. Learning platforms: If you're looking for a more structured approach to learning makeup, online learning platforms can be a great option. Websites like Skillshare, Udemy, and Coursera offer courses on a wide range of makeup topics, taught by industry professionals. These courses can help you deepen your understanding of makeup theory, expand your skill set, and even earn certifications to boost your credentials as a makeup artist. By taking advantage of these online resources, you can continue to grow and improve as a makeup artist. Whether you're looking to expand your knowledge, learn new techniques, or stay current on industry trends, the internet has everything you need to take your skills to the next level. So don't be afraid to explore, experiment, and learn – the world of makeup is waiting for you to dive in and make your mark.

Practice and Experimentation: The key to mastering techniques and developing your own style

Practice and Experimentation: The key to mastering techniques and developing your own style In order to truly excel in the art of makeup, practice and experimentation are essential. Just like any other skill, the more you practice, the better you will become. Experimenting with different techniques, colors, and styles will help you discover what works best for you and allow you to develop your own unique style. Practice makes perfect, so make sure to set aside time each day to work on your makeup skills. Start by practicing basic techniques, such as applying foundation and eyeshadow, and then gradually move on to more advanced techniques like contouring and strobing. Don't be afraid to make mistakes – it's all part of the learning process. Experimentation is also key to developing your own style. Try out different looks and techniques to see what you like best. Don't be afraid to step out of your comfort zone and try something new. You never know – you may discover a new technique or style that you absolutely love. Remember, makeup is an art form, and there are no rules. The most important thing is to have fun and express yourself creatively. By practicing regularly and experimenting with different techniques, you will not only improve your skills but also develop your own unique style that sets you apart from the rest. So go ahead, grab your brushes and makeup palettes, and start practicing and experimenting. The more you practice and experiment, the closer you will be to mastering the art of makeup and becoming a true professional.

Passion and Dedication: The essential ingredient for success in a professional makeup career

Passion and Dedication: The essential ingredient for success in a professional makeup career Passion and dedication are two key factors that can make or break a professional makeup artist's career. In a field as competitive and ever-changing as the beauty industry, it is vital to have a deep love for makeup and a strong commitment to honing your craft in order to succeed. To truly excel in this profession, you must be willing to put in the hard work and long hours necessary to perfect your skills. This means continuously practicing and experimenting with different techniques, staying up-to-date on the latest trends and products, and seeking out opportunities for further education and training. Passion is what drives you to push yourself beyond your limits, to take risks and try new things, and to always strive for excellence in your work. It is what sets you apart from the rest and allows you to create truly unique and inspiring looks for your clients. Dedication, on the other hand, is what keeps you going when the going gets tough. It is the unwavering commitment to your craft, even when faced with challenges or setbacks. Dedication means showing up every day ready to give it your all, and never settling for mediocrity. Together, passion and dedication are the essential ingredients for success in a professional makeup career. With these two qualities as your guiding principles, you can achieve great things in this competitive and rewarding industry. So, if you are truly passionate about makeup and dedicated to becoming the best artist you can be, then the sky is the limit for your career. Embrace your love for beauty and commit yourself fully to your craft, and you will undoubtedly find success and fulfillment in the world of professional makeup.